Unplug
and Unwind

Unplug and Unwind

MINDFUL WAYS TO REST, RELAX, AND FEEL RENEWED

CICO BOOKS

LONDON NEW YORK

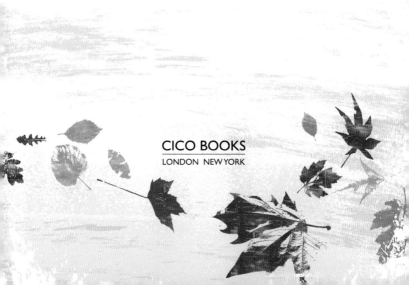

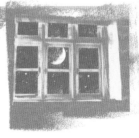

Published in 2024 by CICO Books
An imprint of Ryland Peters & Small Ltd
20–21 Jockey's Fields   341 E 116th St
London WC1R 4BW   New York, NY 10029

www.rylandpeters.com

10 9 8 7 6 5 4 3 2 1

A CIP catalog record for this book is available from the
Library of Congress and the British Library.

ISBN: 978-1-80065-306-1

Printed in China

Illustrations pages 119, 120 and 122–125 by Stephen Dew
All other illustrations by Clare Nicholas

Commissioning editor: Kristine Pidkameny
Senior designer: Emily Breen
Art director: Sally Powell
Head of production: Patricia Harrington
Publishing manager: Penny Craig

Contents

Introduction 6

CHAPTER 1

Rest and Sleep Well 8

CHAPTER 2

Relax into Calm and Happiness 58

CHAPTER 3

Renew with Time to Thrive 98

Text credits 142

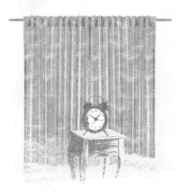

"The beginning is always today."

Mary Shelley

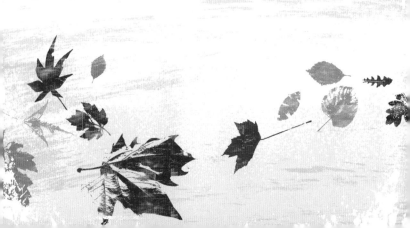

Introduction

In this increasingly digital age, with our constant connection to technology and the fast pace of contemporary life, it can be difficult to decompress and slow down. While often necessary to thrive in today's world, being too plugged-in has its downsides. Checking your phone first thing in the morning or during a night of disrupted sleep has become routine. Hours lost mindlessly engaging with online content is par for the course. The constant interruptions calling out for attention abound. Sound familiar? There is a better way to meet the challenges and stress that can easily overwhelm our daily lives.

Studies show that prioritizing rest and relaxation—to occasionally unplug—is vital to physical, emotional, and mental health. Taking time like this invites more ease and energy into your life. And bringing a mindful approach to the unwanted demands that may arise, benefits your total well-being; it can help you relate to situations differently, reduce stress, and reconnect with being more alive.

The three sections in this book offer a wide variety of mindful ways to rest, relax and renew. Discover how to reset your lifestyle, including to feel more rested if you're having trouble sleeping, tune into your breathing regularly to relax, and explore your senses to experience renewed energy and pleasure. With this inspiring compendium of simple ideas and mindful guidance, you can shift from doing to being and find more balance, calm, and happiness in your life.

CHAPTER 1

Rest and Sleep Well

The Power of Rest

Resting restores us in so many ways and is just as important as the active parts of our day. And while sleep is so important—it helps us heal and regenerate more efficiently, enables our brain to function better, and keeps our moods and blood sugar more stable—it shouldn't be the only time we rest. Here are some tips for building regular breaks for resting into your day:

The 90/10 rule: While working, commit yourself to a 10-minute break every 90 minutes. Do something you enjoy that doesn't require using a computer or phone (playing music is allowed). Take a walk, stare out of the window, do some stretches or breathing exercises, have a snack, or pamper yourself with a face spray or some hand lotion. Repeat throughout your day.

Meditation: Everyone can find a way to meditate that works for them—even if they don't call it that. You can do a walking meditation, a visualization, repeat a mantra, sit and do breathing exercises, or use mindfulness techniques. Choose your own adventure and mix it up. When you're tired and depleted, even just five minutes lying down and breathing mindfully can restore you. There are many different meditation techniques, but the goal is to observe your thoughts and eventually calm the mind by separating yourself from your thoughts.

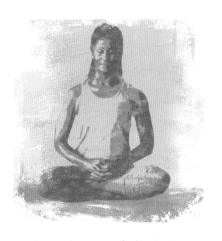

Mindfulness: One way of being more meditative is through mindfulness. This is the act of bringing your attention to the present moment. You can do this by focusing on your breathing or checking in with all your senses. What do you hear, see, feel, smell, and taste? You can try a mindful breathing practice, a body scan, or simply go about your everyday chores more mindfully—for example, be more present when you're washing the dishes or doing the ironing. Or you might be more attentive in your self-care—for example, being more mindful as you wash your hair and body in the shower and enjoying the sensation of the water, rather than mentally running through your to-do list. Mindfulness can be used as part of a meditation practice to quiet the mind.

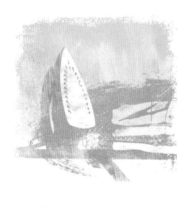

Screen-free time: Screen time does not count as rest. In addition to taking 10 minutes in between working stints, build in screen-free time at the beginning and end of your day. Set your phone to dim all the apps and stay on quiet mode between 8pm and 9am. It's an easy reminder to put the phone down after dinner and until breakfast. This time will help you to be more creative, connect more easily with your partner, and get better sleep.

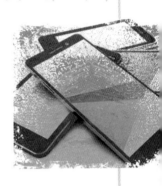

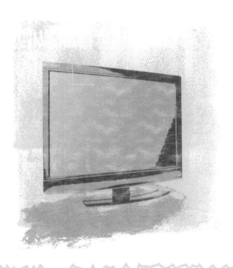

The Importance of Sleep

We spend about a quarter to a third of our lives asleep, but just because we are not awake doesn't mean that time is unproductive. The physiological changes that occur when we are asleep determine how well we feel and perform when we are awake.

It's often said that diet, exercise, and sleep are the three foundational pillars to good health and well-being. While many of us understand the importance of eating a healthy, balanced diet and of keeping fit, we are perhaps less familiar with how important sleep is.

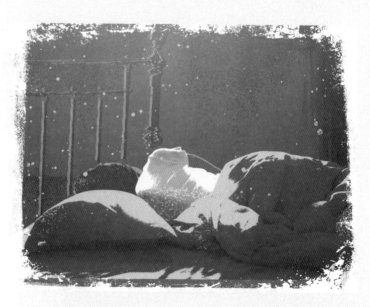

We've all experienced the effects of too little sleep: what it means for our mood, focus, and concentration, and also how it affects us physically—we have less energy and feel tired and groggy. However, the importance of sleep and the consequences of being sleep-deprived go beyond this.

Sleep influences all the major systems in our body, and those systems in turn influence our sleep. Insufficient sleep can disrupt bodily functions that affect how we think and behave, and how we think and behave can disrupt our sleep. Therefore, problems with sleeping can quickly become a vicious cycle.

At its simplest, sleep plays an important role in:

- Creating a healthy immune system

- Repairing muscle

- Consolidating learning and memory

- Regulating growth and appetite through the release of certain hormones

- Regulating mood and emotion.

Sufficient sleep is essential to our well-being, both physically and emotionally, so it is not surprising that when we are deprived of it, we feel the impact in all areas of our life. There is plenty of evidence that poor-quality or too little sleep can have serious consequences for our physical and mental health.

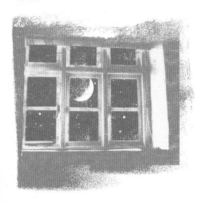

Yawn

Go ahead and give in to that yawn at the end of the day. When you pay attention to your yawn, you may realize just how good it feels—it activates the soothing part of your nervous system, releases feel-good hormones like oxytocin and serotonin, and helps you feel more relaxed. In fact, just reading this probably makes you want to yawn ... so go ahead!

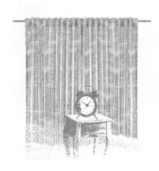

Letting Go

This is a good practice to do lying down, perhaps before you fall asleep or if you wake in the night. Remember that whenever we do these practices, we are not doing them with a particular outcome in mind—you may fall asleep, but also you may not, and that's okay. If you expect to fall asleep and then don't, you will most likely feel frustrated, disappointed, and more, and that is counterproductive. It will only fuel anxiety, which will feed the wakefulness.

1 If you are doing this lying down, begin by becoming aware of the whole body. Notice where it is in contact with the bed or mat and how that feels—soft? Hard? (You can do the practice sitting if you prefer.)

2 Take a deep breath in and let it out suddenly (if you make a noise as you exhale, that's okay). Do this two or three times, noticing as you do so how the body softens and lets go as you breathe out.

3 Begin tuning into the out-breath. Notice how the body relaxes and softens—perhaps be curious about which parts of the body feel loose. Just let go.

4 You may notice a feeling of "holding on" or tension in a particular part of the body, perhaps in the face or the torso. Simply acknowledge that tension is here. You may experience a letting go, but there is no need to force anything.

5 Every time the mind wanders, bring it back.

Focus on the Body

When we are lying awake, it is very easy to become caught up in a thought spiral about not sleeping: Why we can't sleep, how it's affecting us, and all the associated emotions these thoughts create. It is helpful if we can shift from a sense of needing to do something about not being able to sleep, to practicing simply being as we are—which, in this moment, is awake. We can do this by making the body our focus. This might be a part of the body, such as the breath, the whole body, or, as in the following practice, an exploration of the outline of the body.

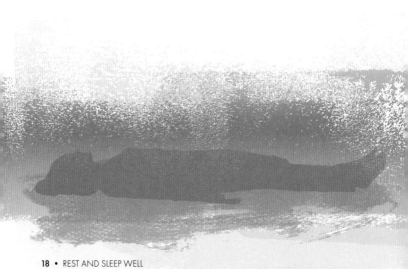

Outlining the Body

Although this is a lying-down practice, remember to let go of any
expectation that you will fall asleep.

1 In your mind's eye, begin outlining the body, as if you were drawing
around it. Then begin moving your attention across the contours of the
body, for example around and across the top of the feet, the belly, the
chest, and the head. Always maintain an awareness of any points of
contact with the bed, and mentally draw around them.

2 Notice any physical sensations, such as touch and temperature,
or internal sensations, such as tingling or numbness. Do not expect to
feel anything in particular, or to have a specific experience. Simply
connect with this body, lying here in this moment.

3 Every time you become aware of the mind wandering, acknowledge
it as "thinking" and gently bring your attention back to outlining the
body. Do this over and over again. It is the nature of the mind to wander,
and you are training yourself to notice it wandering and bring it back
to a focus, in this case, the body. It is important that you don't give
yourself a hard time when your mind wanders. We can't stop thinking,
but we can learn to choose where we want to place our attention,
whether on our thoughts or on the body. In this practice, choose always
to bring our attention back to the body.

4 Continue in this way as long as you wish. You may fall asleep,
or you may "fall awake." There is no goal, and if you happen to
fall asleep, that is a bonus.

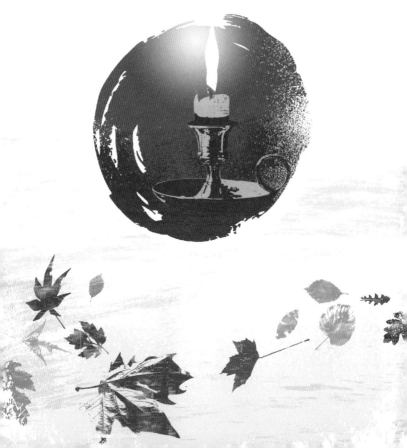

"Sleep is that golden chain that ties health and our bodies together."

Thomas Dekker

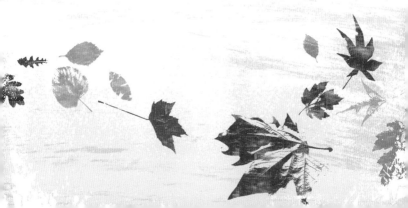

How Sleep Is Regulated

The body has a built-in system called the circadian rhythm, which is responsible for regulating sleepiness and wakefulness over a 24-hour period (the time it takes for the Earth to circle the sun). The circadian rhythm usually emerges between two and six months after birth. It is controlled by the area of the brain that responds to light and receives input direct from the retina in the eye. It causes wakefulness to fluctuate through the day, and then, as darkness falls, it encourages sleepiness.

If we go to bed and rise at a regular time, we will help ourselves create and maintain a balanced circadian rhythm. It is easily disrupted by changes in

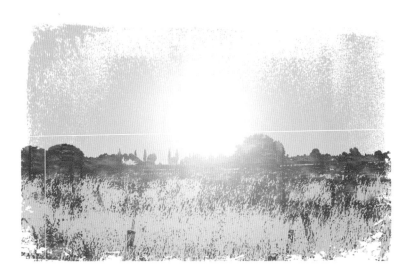

sleeping or waking patterns, perhaps caused by shift work, late nights at weekends, traveling across time zones, stress, or illness. We can strengthen our circadian rhythm by following good sleeping habits.

Our circadian rhythm can change over time. When we are younger, we are more likely to be "night owls," staying up and rising later, and as we get older, we are more likely to go to bed and rise earlier. The circadian rhythm plays a role in some important systems that influence our sleeping habits, such as how much melatonin the body produces. It also regulates our core body temperature, so that it increases during the day and drops at night as we fall asleep. This then plays a role in helping us to stay asleep (hence the importance of maintaining a cool room). Our temperature usually begins to rise again at about 4am, as we start to move from sleep to waking.

TIP

To avoid an elevated body temperature at bedtime, if you are exercising, do so at least 4 hours before going to bed. Likewise, the best time for taking a hot bath is about 60–90 minutes before bedtime. It is not the raised body temperature from the bath that makes us sleepy, but the subsequent drop as we cool down.

A Morning Walk

The dark of night and light of day are determined by the Earth's rotation around the sun, and our circadian rhythm is linked to these natural cycles. We can help to strengthen or reset a disrupted circadian rhythm by exposing ourselves to light (indoors or out), which will signal to the brain that it is day and time to wake up. A morning walk will energize us and help to reset a disrupted circadian rhythm, and it can also be an opportunity for some mindfulness practice.

TIP

Take a walk first thing—it could be on the way to work or simply a stroll through a local park or around the block. To make the walk a practice, walk, and know that you are walking. You don't need to walk more slowly than usual but do pay attention to what is arising. Avoid the temptation to put on your headphones, check your cellphone, or email as you are walking.

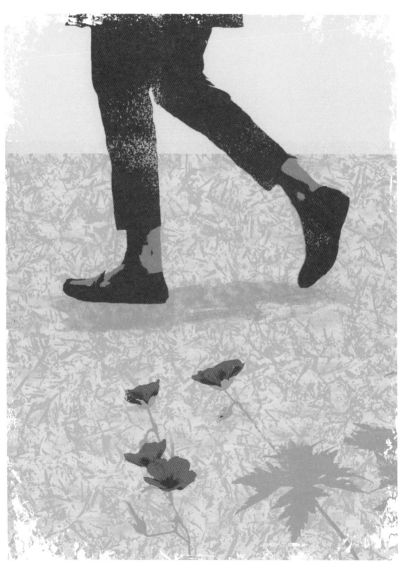

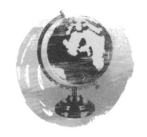

Do something today
that your future self
will thank you for.

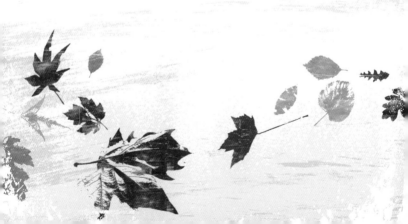

Mindful Walking

1 Begin by dropping your attention to the soles of your feet. Notice that sense of contact and how the sensations shift as the pressure varies from toe to heel and from one foot to the other.

2 You may choose to tune into your breathing as you walk, noticing the in-breath and the out-breath while maintaining awareness of your feet on the ground.

3 After a while, you may want to expand your attention to become aware of the rest of the body: the legs, torso, arms, and head. Continue to expand your attention to become aware of the environment—the sights, sounds, and smells around you.

4 If you have time and feel comfortable doing so, you may choose to stop and stand still (you could do this as you wait to cross a street, for example). Soak up the morning light, perhaps experience a sense of warmth on the body, or of cold air touching the skin. Open up to the sounds of nature—the birdsong, the breeze in the trees, or perhaps the buzz of traffic and people around you.

5 When you are ready, continue walking. This practice can be as long or as short as you wish. Give yourself the gift of this time for yourself before you enter the busy day ahead.

If you can't go outside, try this practice indoors by walking across a room. Open the drapes, and look out the window from time to time, drinking in the early-morning light.

How Much Sleep Do We Need?

There is no "golden" number of hours that is the perfect amount of sleep, and subjective sleep quality (whether we feel we have had a good night's sleep or not) is as significant as duration. Two people can sleep for a similar amount of time with similar periods of wakefulness, and yet perceive it very differently.

In general, eight hours is usually about right for adults; children and young adults will need more and the elderly less. However, it is important not to get too hooked on numbers, particularly if you do have trouble sleeping, since there may be a tendency to constantly measure how you are doing and then feel disappointed if you are falling short. This may create additional anxiety about sleeping, and that is unhelpful. Mindfulness helps us to let go of expectations and of striving toward a particular goal, and instead helps us to be okay with the way things are.

Ask yourself the following questions after an average night's sleep:

- Do I feel healthy and happy?

- Do I depend on caffeine to get through the day (particularly first thing in the morning)?

- Do I feel sleepy during the day? (This is usually a sign that you are not getting enough sleep.)

Depending on your answers, you may decide to make sleep a priority in your life.

Your Ideal Amount of Sleep

Try to work out the number of hours' sleep that is best for you by sleeping for a particular length of time and waking naturally (without an alarm) feeling refreshed, without needing any stimulants such as caffeine. However, you may want to have an alarm clock set as a back-up!

1 Pay off any sleep debt by getting plenty of sleep. You may need to do this while you're on vacation!

2 Using 7½ hours as a starting point, count back from the time you need to get up and make that your bedtime (factor in a short period of "falling-asleep time").

3 Begin going to bed at that time for at least a week or, better still, ten days, and notice whether you begin waking up just before your alarm.

4 If after ten days you still need the alarm, go to bed a little earlier and continue until you find the right duration for you.

If you have the flexibility to get up at any time, another option is to go to bed at the same time each night and notice when you wake up naturally, without any outside interference. Doing this over a period of a couple weeks will allow you to determine how much sleep you personally need.

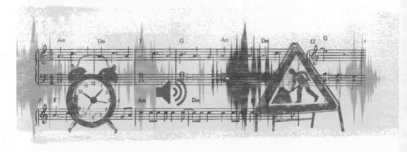

What Happens When We Don't Get Enough Sleep?

Many people don't realize that sleep is one of the cornerstones of well-being, along with diet and exercise. We may be aware that regularly eating junk food and not exercising affects our physical and mental well-being, but we may not make the same connection with not getting enough sleep. Although this is an emerging field in research, with new discoveries being made all the time, it is known that sleep is closely linked to all the body's physiological systems, and so when sleep is disrupted, it is inevitable that we don't function at our best, emotionally, mentally, and physically.

Emotions and mood

We have all experienced how we become more irritable and reactive when we are lacking sleep and there is usually a decline in mood as well. We are more likely to rate our mood negatively after one night of sleep deprivation. Laboratory studies suggest that when we are deprived of sleep, we may become more intolerant of and frustrated with others, more likely to blame others for hypothetical predicaments, and less likely to compromise to find a mutually satisfying outcome. We also lack empathy and are more self-centered.

The brain and performance

Lack of sleep particularly affects basic attention and vigilance, the cornerstones for more complex thinking. The ability to maintain sustained attention is also critical in many industries where work involves monitoring, so poor sleep can have an impact on safety as well as performance.

Most of us begin to experience slower reactions and responses after we have been awake for 16 hours, and this increases as wakefulness persists. Even restricting sleep by a couple of hours in a night can lead to significant lengthening of reaction times. If we sleep six hours a night for two weeks, our performance will be impaired to the same degree as if we had been awake for 48 hours non-stop.

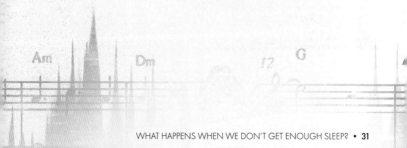

Our ability to learn new things and remember them is essential for basic survival as well as performance. Sleep is crucial in preparing the brain to acquire new information before learning, and it also plays an essential role afterward, consolidating learning and integrating it into long-term memory banks, from where it can be retrieved when it is needed. If these two stages are disrupted by sleep deprivation, the development of new memories—and therefore learning—will be hindered. Next time you are studying for an exam, starting a new job, or learning a new skill, invest in your sleep before and after to help you get the most out of it.

The emotional content of memories is also affected by sleep deprivation. It appears that positive and neutral memories are more susceptible than negative memories, so if we are deprived of sleep our positive and neutral memories are more likely to be degraded and lost. That leaves us with a preponderance of negative memories. As human beings, we already have a natural negativity bias in our thinking, which is tied to our essential survival wiring—it is more important to remember where a potential threat is located than the experience of watching a beautiful sunrise. People who practice mindfulness often comment on how they begin to notice the small positive experiences that occur throughout the day, but that are commonly missed in the distractions of daily life. This helps counteract the natural negativity bias. Once we consciously notice a happy experience, it becomes banked into our long-term memory.

Obesity

People who haven't had enough sleep have reduced levels of the hormone leptin, which is responsible for suppressing appetite, and an increase in the peptide ghrelin, which stimulates it. Therefore, chronic sleep deprivation may cause us to eat more and gain weight. It may also cause us to make unhealthy food choices. In addition, if we are overweight, we are more likely to have problems sleeping. Sleep apnea can increase the risk of obesity. The excessive sleepiness caused by apnea inhibits the desire to exercise, which contributes to being overweight.

Immune system and pain

"Sleep is the best medicine" is not an old wives' tale. The proper functioning of the body's immune system is compromised by poor sleep. A good night's sleep is essential when battling acute infection, but sleep can be disrupted by pain and illness, which in turn can delay healing. There is an association between lack of sleep and an increase in spontaneous pain, as well as general physical discomfort, headaches, and muscle and stomach pain.

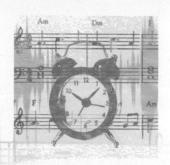

Sleep Deprivation

When we are sleep deprived:

- We become more easily distracted, and for longer periods

- The brain is not primed for learning and is unable to consolidate effectively what is learned, thereby affecting long-term memory

- We experience an increasingly negative bias in mood and memory

- Our appetite increases, so we eat more and make unhealthier choices

- Our energy levels drop and so we exercise less

- We experience pain more acutely

- Our immune system is compromised

- Essential hormones go out of kilter, which can affect growth, reproduction, and other bodily functions, along with the metabolism of glucose, which can lead to diabetes.

These negative effects often remain even when alertness and vigilance are restored with stimulants such as caffeine. Therefore, although we may feel more awake and alert, behind the scenes the body's systems are not functioning at their best or even properly.

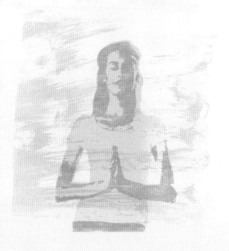

Practicing mindfulness should not be seen as a means of getting by with less sleep, but rather about waking up so that we are more likely to notice how our behavior and performance change when we are sleep deprived— and can then do something about it. That might mean not putting ourselves or others at risk by doing certain tasks such as driving when sleepy or simply acknowledging that when we are over-tired, we will be more reactive and less tolerant of others, as well as doing what we can to address our lack of sleep.

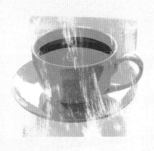

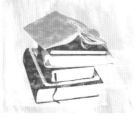

Developing Awareness

1 As you are reading about sleep deprivation, what are you noticing about your response to it? First take a moment to become aware of the story that is playing out in your head, noticing any emotions arising or felt sensations in the body. Notice if you are catastrophizing about what you are reading and thinking of the long-term consequences of not getting enough sleep; or perhaps you feel a sense of recognition or familiarity—ah, that's why I do that! It can be reassuring to know that our behavior is a consequence of the body's systems being out of kilter. As always, bring a sense of friendly interest to this reflection.

2 Now reflect on how your mood and emotions are usually affected by not getting enough sleep. How about your performance and the way you interact with others? Are you more reactive and less compassionate toward others?

If you are not sure, then just start doing this type of reflection at different times—when you are fresh and awake as well as tired and sleepy—and notice how your performance, mood, and relationships with others may be affected.

3 Remember that there is no need to be critical about what you discover, but instead bring an attitude of curiosity and self-compassion to the experiment and simply acknowledge how things are. This is about becoming familiar with our habitual patterns and bringing them into awareness. Doing this can help us spot them earlier so they become useful "red flags," warning us that perhaps things are out of kilter, and we need to take some wise action.

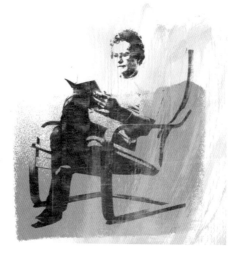

The Effect of Technology

For most of us, the days when bedrooms were simply places to sleep and make love are long gone. First it was the appearance of the television, then the smartphone, laptop, e-reader, and tablet. All are now commonplace in our bedrooms. There is nothing wrong with the technology or the objects themselves. It's simply that the presence of these items immediately signals activity—doing something—rather than resting or letting go of activity. Also, the way we engage with them can have a negative impact on our sleep.

A smartphone, laptop, tablet, or television screen acts as a mini sun, emitting blue light that interferes with the production of melatonin that is essential for becoming sleepy. While on some phones it is possible to activate a nighttime filter that reduces the blue light, it doesn't remove it entirely.

The gadgets themselves are a source of distraction. Checking emails and status updates on social media keeps us in a state of hyperarousal. The brain remains on alert for what might pop into our inbox or social media feed, rather than being encouraged to wind down in preparation for sleep.

Using a smartphone for work keeps us connected mentally long after we have physically left the office. It becomes harder to disconnect from work during the evening, and that can lead to rumination that disrupts sleep. If you work from home, it is even more important to give yourself a mental break by making a clear distinction between work and leisure hours.

Notifications and alerts can interrupt our sleep. Healthy sleepers will experience up to ten brief arousals or awakenings per hour of sleep. These usually last only seconds, and they are often associated with body movement. Their fleeting nature means they are usually forgotten, and so we are unaware

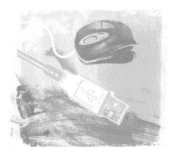

of them unless they are prolonged because of a sound or other factor such as smell. If an alert sounds on your phone during one of these mini awakenings, you are more likely to wake up properly. If you are someone who experiences problems with sleeping, this can set off the reactive pattern of insomnia.

Practice Noticing

Next time you find yourself catastrophizing about being awake when you'd rather be sleeping, notice how you are relating to being awake. What are you noticing in the head (thoughts), heart (emotions), and body (physical sensations)? There is no need to judge what you find. Simply notice how uncomfortable resisting our experience can be.

Calming the Mind

A traditional suggestion for getting to sleep is to try counting sheep. This practice works in a similar way—if the mind is particularly busy, we can count our breaths as a way of steadying our attention and moving our attention out of the head (thinking) and into the body.

In this practice, we count to ten and then start again. When you find yourself going beyond 10, simply start again at 1. You can do this practice lying in bed or sitting, in the same way as Paying Attention to the Breath (see page 67).

1 2 3 4 5 6 7 8 9 10

TIP

Sleeping in a cooler room is helpful in facilitating the natural drop in body temperature that will encourage the onset of sleep.

Counting Breaths

1 Whether sitting or lying down, check your posture. Begin to tune into your breathing. Notice how the breath is made up of an in-breath and an out-breath. For counting purposes, both of these make up one whole breath.

2 Every time you breathe in and out, count 1. Continue up to 10 and then start again.

3 Don't worry if you lose count or go beyond 10. As soon as you realize, simply return to 1. Continue for as long or short a time as you like.

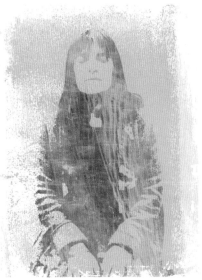

Just Three Things

When we begin practicing mindfulness, we soon learn how helpful it is to turn our attention to the body. By cultivating an attitude of curiosity about what is arising physically in the body, we are able to shift our attention from our head,

Temperature, Touch, Breath

1 Lie flat on your back with your legs outstretched, your feet falling away, and your arms at your side. Turn your hands palm up.

2 **Temperature:** Notice any part of the body that feels warm and explore what the sensation of warmth is like. Can you notice different degrees of warmth? Is there a point at which warm becomes hot? Notice how you are responding to what you find—does it feel positive, negative, or neutral (simply noticing without judging).

3 Let go of warmth, and now notice any part of the body that feels cool or cold. Explore internally and externally in the same way as for warmth and heat, again noticing how you respond.

4 **Touch:** Letting go of temperature, turn your attention to touch. Notice any points of contact with the mattress (the heels, the thighs, the shoulders ...). Notice how the contact feels (hard, soft, welcoming, resisting ...). What else is touching: fabric in contact with skin, skin

which is often busy overthinking the latest drama in our lives. There are many body-focused practices to explore; this one is particularly simple and therefore ideal if you are lying awake in bed. Just accept whatever happens. You may fall asleep, and you may not. The intention is simply to be present to whatever arises moment by moment. In this practice, we focus our attention on just three things, one after the other: Temperature, touch, and breath.

on skin ... how many different types of contact can you identify?
Explore touch.

5 Breath: Letting go of touch, narrow your attention to focus solely on your breathing. Notice whether it is slow and deep, or short and shallow, or if it varies. There is no need to change your breathing or try to breathe in a particular way; simply allow the breath to breathe itself. You might begin by focusing on the part of the body where you feel the breath most strongly (the chest or belly), but as your attention becomes focused, notice where else in the body you are experiencing breathing. Become aware of movement, rhythm, rising, falling, expanding, contracting ...

6 When you are ready, expand your attention to the whole body, noticing the temperature, sensations of touch, and breath entering and leaving the body.

Sleep Like a Baby

Sleep is on the top of the heap of what we need to be healthy and to perform at optimum levels. Although some people who are chronically sleep deprived may be high functioning, for most of us mood, focus, and overall joy factor are negatively affected by persistent lack of sleep. Health professionals agree that sleep deprivation is a serious health concern and a growing global problem. Technology, caffeine abuse, the pace of the world, financial concerns, illness, and anxiety are a few of the thieves in the night that come to steal our slumber.

It's hard not to envy the sleep of a baby—what is it that they know that we don't? Or maybe it's what they don't know! They don't have jobs, children to take care of, world peace to worry about, or saving the environment on their minds. It is possible to get back to this state of inner freedom, but we have to prepare the mind and body. A little sleep hygiene can create the right conditions to pave the way to sleeping like a baby, every night.

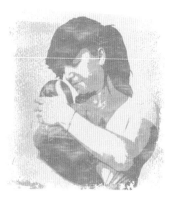

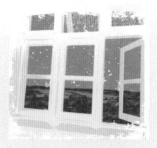

Sleep Hygiene

Here are a few ways to soothe the savage nighttime beasties and get a good night's rest. Test this prescription for a week at least.

- Turn off screens 30 minutes to one hour before bed. Instead, read something uplifting (or very tedious and boring!) Avoid the news.

- Keep the lights low.

- Take a bath.

- Use essential oils, such as lavender, on the bottoms of your feet.

- Drink chamomile tea or Golden Milk (see page 48), 30 minutes before bed.

- Keep the window slightly open for air circulation.

- Keep a gratitude journal at your bedside.

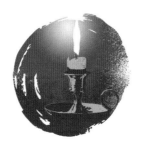

I lay my mind to rest and welcome peaceful release into my body.

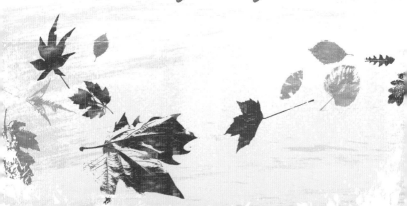

Focus on the Breath

If you usually have trouble falling asleep, Bee Breath (*Bhramari Pranayama*) is wonderful for relieving stress and sends a healing vibration through the vocal cords and chest. It can be practiced seated—on a chair, sitting up in bed, or sitting cross-legged on the floor (either flat on the ground or on a bolster or folded blanket so you are slightly elevated)—or lying down.

Bee Breath

Place one hand on your heart and one hand on your belly (or you might like to put your index fingers in your ears with your elbows pointing down, as this position is especially helpful for sleep trouble). Inhale and as you exhale make a deep humming sound like a bee. Hum from the chest and belly more than from the lips. Do not strain for the sound to last—rather, let it softly and naturally fade in the way a buzz from a bee fades as it flies farther away from you. Practice 5–10 rounds.

Golden Milk

A warm, soothing drink before bedtime can help you to relax and unwind as you prepare for sleep. Golden Milk also has many health benefits—in particular, it's great for joints and reducing inflammation.

You can buy Golden Milk, but it's easier and cheaper to make a batch at home that will last a few days. To make a batch of Golden Milk, simply double or triple the quantities as required. The milk will keep for 3–5 days, stored in an airtight container in the refrigerator. Reheat in a saucepan on the stove or in the microwave.

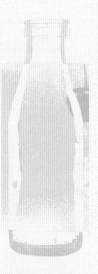

TIP

Note: If you cannot obtain whole spices, you can substitute ground spices: ¼ teaspoon of ground cloves, ¼ teaspoon ground cinnamon, and ⅛ teaspoon ground cardamom. In this case, there is no need to boil the spices in water first—simply add the ground spices to the milk, turmeric, pepper, and oil.

½ cup (120ml) of water

4–8 whole cloves

1 small cinnamon stick

3–6 green cardamom pods

1 cup (240ml) milk of your choice, such as cow's milk,
almond, soy, coconut, or hemp

½ teaspoon ground turmeric

¼ teaspoon freshly ground black pepper

½–1 teaspoon pure extra virgin coconut oil or almond oil
(omit this if using coconut milk)

1 teaspoon raw honey or stevia, to taste

MAKES 1 SERVING

Put the water in a small saucepan and add the cloves, cinnamon stick,
and cardamom pods. Bring to a boil for 3–5 minutes. Add the milk, ground
turmeric, pepper, and oil to the saucepan and simmer on low for about
7 minutes, stirring occasionally with a whisk, but do not let it boil. Strain and
serve. Add the raw honey or stevia if desired. Let cool before drinking.

Herbal Infusions

Infusions are derived from the more fragile parts of plants, which include the bud, flower, leaves, and scent-producing parts. These delicate herbs require steeping rather than boiling or simmering. They release their flavor more quickly than tougher roots and barks.

The proportion of water to herb and the required time to infuse varies greatly, depending on the herb. Start out with the below proportions and then experiment. The more herb you use and the longer you let it steep, the stronger the brew. Let your intuition and taste preference be your guide.

1 tablespoon herbs of your choice, such as chamomile, lemon balm, passionflower, valerian, lavender, or thyme

1 cup (240ml) water

MAKES 1 SERVING

Add the herbs to a heat-resistant glass bowl. Boil the water in a teakettle, pour it over the herbs, and let steep for 30–60 minutes. Strain into a mug, then enjoy either at room temperature or reheated.

Deep Sleep
Herbal Immersion

Immersing yourself in a warm, aromatic bath about 60–90 minutes before bedtime is optimum for encouraging a good nights' sleep. This combination of herbs provides calming scents that will help you to relax.

1 cup (240g) Epsom salts

1 cup (240g) baking soda (bicarbonate of soda)

12 drops clary sage essential oil

12 drops lavender essential oil

8 drops jasmine essential oil

MAKES 4 PORTIONS

Combine the Epsom salts and baking soda in a mixing bowl with a wooden spoon and then add the essential oils and blend well. Store in a sealable jar or canister and add a few drops to your nighttime bath as needed.

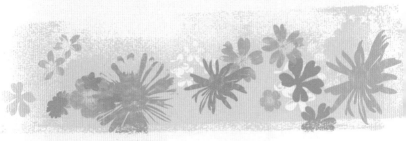

A Soothing Nighttime Bath

The oils in this recipe are thought to be beneficial for relaxation and sleeplessness. See page 94 for more information about essential oils.

2–3 tablespoons (30–45ml) liquid Castile soap
(or you can use vegetable or jojoba oil!)

2 drops frankincense essential oil

2 drops geranium essential oil

2 drops sandalwood essential oil

2 drops lavender essential oil

MAKES 1 PORTION

Mix together the soap and essential oils in a small bowl. Fill a bathtub with hot water, then add the soap mixture and swirl to mix well. Get into the bath and soak in the water for about 20 minutes.

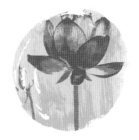

"Put your thoughts
to sleep, do not let them
cast a shadow over the
moon of your heart.
Let go of thinking."

Rumi

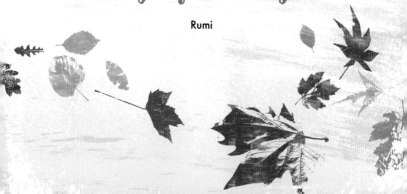

Bedroom Retreat

As it's often the last place you tidy up, take some time today to make your bedroom a nurturing space to retreat to at the end of the day: diffuse some lavender essential oil, light a candle, fluff up your pillows, add a fuzzy blanket to your bed, get a heating pad or hot water bottle, or just clear out the clutter so you can truly relax at the end of your day.

I give myself permission to no longer be on the go.

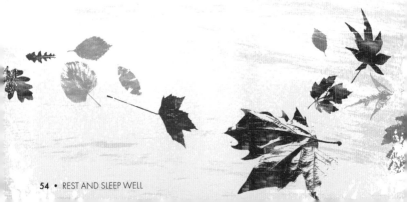

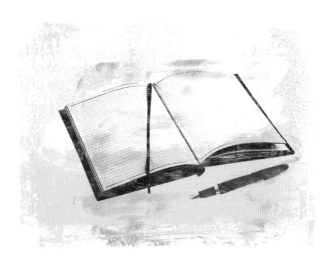

Five Good Things

Before you go to bed, list five good things that happened today.
You can do this in a journal, or simply tick them off on your fingers.
Even the smallest win counts!

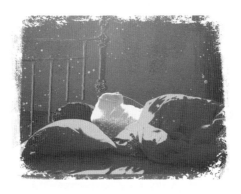

Bedtime Massage

Give your hard-working body a bit of love before bed—rub some
lotion or essential oils on your hands and feet, massage your temples
and cheeks and jaw, and gently tend to any aching muscles.
Place a warm lavender compress on your forehead, snuggle up
to a heating pad, and take a few soothing deep breaths.

Sleep as Surrender

As you climb into bed tonight, remember that sleep is a powerful lesson in surrender: we don't know when and how we will slide from wakefulness into slumber, but we know it will happen. All we can do is create the proper conditions, and then lie down and trust.

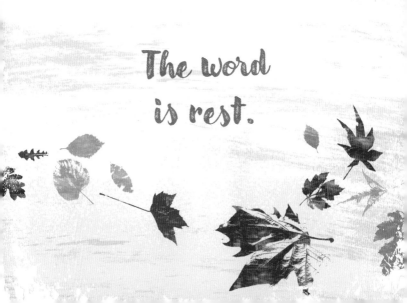

The word
is rest.

CHAPTER 2

Relax into Calm and Happiness

The Art of Relaxation

Sometimes we feel helpless when things are difficult. After honestly acknowledging the reality of the situation and how we feel about it we may realize that we can't fix it or make it better. At this point, we can ask "What do I need right now?" This could be something that will bring you a sense of calm, like attention to your breath or taking the time to appreciate yourself and feel inner happiness.

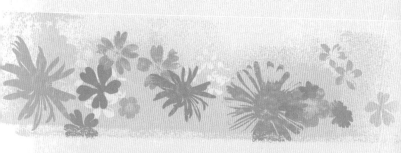

Smile a Little Smile

Everything you need to be happy today or in the future lies within you right now. Wishing you were someone else with other talents and skills, or regretting that you did or didn't make a certain decision, will take you further away from happiness. Looking yourself in the eye and appreciating who you are, with all your beauty, skills, and potential, will take you to wherever you have the determination to be.

When we are anxious or stressed, we tense up—often in the shoulders, the jaw, or around the forehead. There is a sense of tightening. We can practice cultivating the opposite by softening inside. Imagine you are smiling inside. The lips soften, the throat opens, and there is a sense of release. You can take this further by intentionally making eye contact and smiling at people you meet. Can you smile inside today?

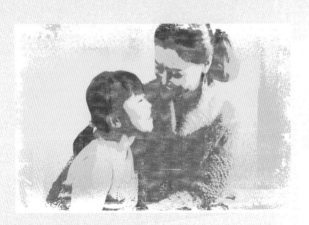

Feet on the Floor

This is one of the simplest and most useful practices to do when things are feeling difficult. When we are stressed, our breath becomes shallow and fast, making it difficult to turn our attention to the breath: the breath may feel elusive and awareness of this only makes us feel worse. When we feel like this, the best thing we can do is to ground ourselves by connecting with the earth beneath us. We can do this most easily through our feet.

When something is weighted at the bottom, it is unlikely to fall over. Focusing your attention on your feet on the floor is like weighting yourself so you don't fall over. You instantly bring yourself into contact with the present moment. The sense of groundlessness eases off. Whatever is going on is still there, but you are able to face it from a place of stability and strength.

Feel Your Feet

Turn your attention to the feet. Do it now. Feel the sensations of your feet in contact with the floor. Push down slightly through the bottom of the feet. It is as if your feet were glued to the floor. The ground is solid beneath your feet, perhaps you can feel your shoes or socks. Explore these sensations. Wiggle your toes if you'd like to.

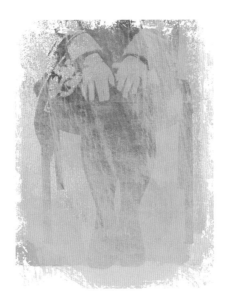

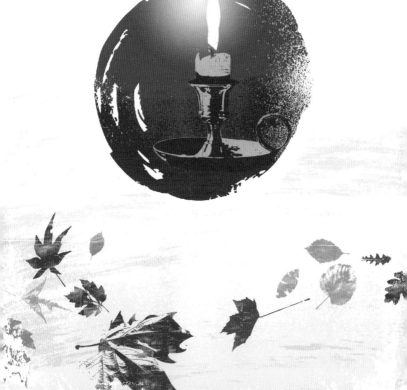

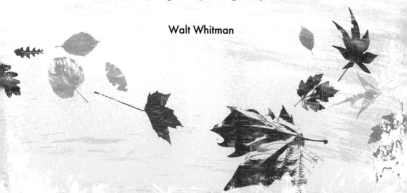

"Happiness not in another place but this place ... not for another hour, but this hour."

Walt Whitman

Exhale

When you breathe in, you activate the body's sympathetic nervous system (the "activating" and energizing part of the nervous system), and when you breathe out, you activate the parasympathetic nervous system, the so-called "relaxation response" of the body. One way to take advantage of the soothing effects of the out-breath is to lengthen your exhale deliberately; for example, you can breathe in for four counts, and then breathe out for six counts. When you need a moment of soothing today, take a deep breath in and really linger on the exhale.

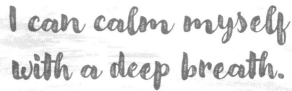

I can calm myself with a deep breath.

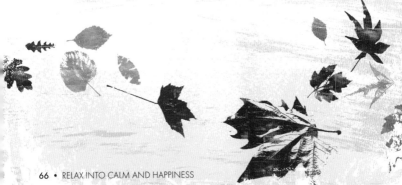

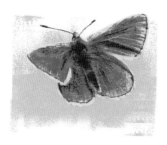

Paying Attention
to the Breath

The breath is a great object to focus our attention on: It is accessible and because it is a moving target, we must exert some effort to keep paying attention to it. The breath also changes according to our frame of mind. If we are anxious, we may find ourselves breathing faster and shallower or perhaps even holding the breath, whereas when we are relaxed, we usually breathe more slowly and deeply.

How is your breath right now? Simply drop your attention into the chest or belly and begin to notice it, becoming aware of its characteristics. There is no need to change it or breathe in a particular way (such as inhaling and exhaling through the nose instead of the mouth, or vice versa). By tuning into the breath regularly, we can become familiar with our "normal" state and any patterns that may arise according to how we are feeling.

We can also do this as a more formal meditation practice by following the steps described on the following pages.

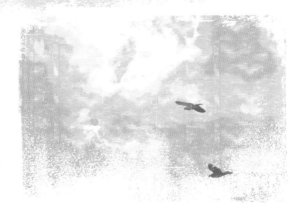

Breath Awareness

1 Find a place where you won't be disturbed and check your posture. Begin by becoming aware of the breath. Where are you feeling it most strongly? This may be in the belly, in the chest, or around the nostrils or upper lip. It doesn't matter where it is but make a clear intention to place your attention there. You may want to place a hand on the belly to help connect with the felt sense of breathing.

2 Continue following the breath. Be curious about it. What does it feel like physically in the body? Notice the in-breath, stay with it, and then notice the transition to an out-breath, and then back to an in-breath.

3 Sooner rather than later you will find that your attention is somewhere else—maybe thinking about your to-do list, about a vacation, or about another person. It is the nature of the mind to wander, and all you have to do is acknowledge it and redirect your attention back to the breath. You will find yourself doing this over and over again, and that's okay.

4 Every time you realize your attention has wandered, you are experiencing a moment of awareness. Every time you bring your attention back with an attitude of kindness and gentleness, you are cultivating those qualities toward yourself. It is also helpful to notice what is on your mind, simply as feedback. What is grabbing your attention?

5 Begin by doing this for five minutes or so, then gradually extend the time if you can.

TIP

You can also do this practice more informally, perhaps while sitting on a bus or train, or at your desk. You can do it standing up or lying down. Practice doing it as often as you can in a variety of situations and locations, including at night.

Breathe Deeply

If you are stressed, panicked, or unhappy, you can usually feel yourself
breathing in the top part of your chest. Take a moment to notice your breathing.
Then consciously breathe from the lower part of your abdomen. Slow down
your breathing and see how quickly you start to calm down. Try to make deep
breathing a habit. Be aware of your own breath and take time in your day to
adjust it. If you're having an argument or feeling emotional, literally take a few
deep breaths—remove yourself from the situation to somewhere a bit quieter
and breathe deeply. It really works!

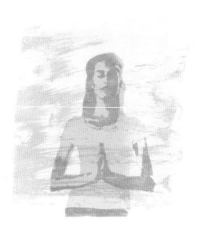

Walk, Knowing That You Are Walking

Walking is a great way to weave mindfulness into your everyday life. There are so many opportunities for practice when we are walking outside and also indoors. You can do it for a few steps or take a mindful walk (see page 27).

Any practice involving movement is also good to do when you are feeling anxious and it is too challenging to stay still. Even simply going barefoot can help to ground you and calm the mind.

Go Barefoot

1 Choose a safe place to walk barefoot and take off your shoes and socks. Indoors, on the grass in your backyard, on sand, in water, or even mud if you are feeling adventurous, are all great places to practice mindfulness.

2 Drop your attention down to the soles of the feet as they lift, shift, and place.

3 Feel the ground through the soles of your feet. Wriggle your toes. Expand your awareness to include the whole body and the environment.

What Pushes Your Buttons Today?

It might be someone cutting in front of you in traffic, a pressing deadline, or a general feeling of being overwhelmed. It might be to do with someone else or perhaps it's the eternal to-do list running through your mind. It may be one thing or a lot of things. Notice who, what, and when—there's no need to worry about why.

Noticing what makes us stressed can help us to develop strategies to manage situations. There are always going to be things that are out of our control but simple changes in behavior can sometimes make a difference. Realizing how much we create our own stress empowers us to take action to reduce it.

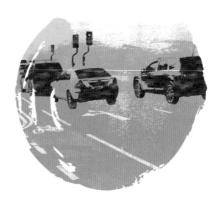

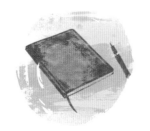

Where attention goes,
energy flows.

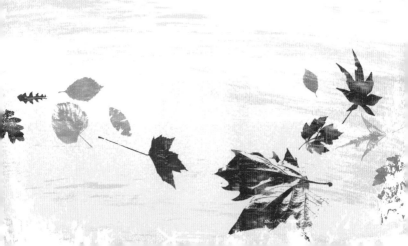

Exploring Resistance

Suffering is often the result of resisting our experience. We don't like the way we are, the way someone else is, or a particular situation, and we wish things were different. Resisting the way things actually are generates a lot of physical tension in the body (as we brace ourselves against what is arising), as well as mental exhaustion (as we try to fix or change what is arising).

If you have trouble sleeping, you will have experienced something like this as you lie in bed. You may feel physically tired, but you are awake and your mind is hyper-alert—worrying about not sleeping, wondering why, thinking about the next day and how you are going to feel more exhausted, and so on and so on. We can feel stuck, going round and round like a hamster on a wheel, and we don't know how to step out of it.

We can't do anything about feeling physically tired; that is how the body is right now. We can however, do something about all the additional layers of suffering we are adding on top of "body tired"—the thoughts about not sleeping and its consequences. That is within our control. Resisting how things are is the problem, therefore the easiest way to relax or let go is to stop trying to make things different.

However, for most of us, stopping trying to make things different is usually something we have to learn how to do—it's not our natural reaction. Whenever we are learning new skills, it is better to begin with something minor that doesn't have a strong emotional charge. The practice on pages 76–77 will help you tune in to your personal experience of resistance, and by doing so, you will find your own route to acceptance.

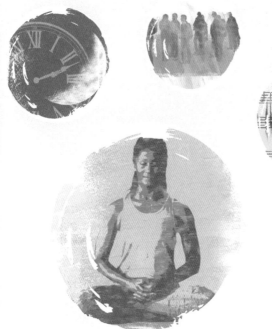

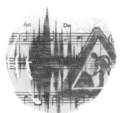

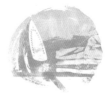

Acknowledging Resistance

Try this practice when something is not right with you. It could be a moment during an unpleasant commute, feeling frustrated as you stand in line when you are in a rush, or when you are late for an appointment and you are being held up in traffic.

1 First of all, be aware that things are not as you would like them to be. This is easier to pick up if you have been doing a body-focused practice such as Paying Attention to the Breath (see page 67) regularly, since usually the first signs we notice are those arising from the body. Perhaps there is tension in the neck or shoulders, maybe we are tapping our feet, drumming our fingers, or clenching our jaw ... each person has their own physical signs of stress.

2 Once you are aware, acknowledge it, saying "Resistance is here" (or words to that effect, such as "Irritation is here"). Acknowledging and naming what is here is the first step toward accepting it.

3 Then tune in to how that resistance or emotion feels in the body. Where are you feeling it? How does it feel: Solid or soft? Is it moving or staying in one place? Are there any sensations associated with it (tingling, pulsing, stabbing ...)? Be curious about how resistance feels. If there are no strong sensations but just a sense of numbness, that is equally interesting: How far does the numbness extend around the body? What can you discover?

4 We are not trying to make the resistance or emotion go away. We are exploring how it feels to be with it—to allow it to be present, since it already is. You could say silently to yourself, "It's okay, let me feel this."

5 We may stay with the physical sensations of the resistance only fleetingly before taking our attention to the breath or breathing through the feet on the floor to anchor ourselves. We may choose to dip back and forth between the breath and the sensations, but only if it feels okay to do so. Stay with the uncomfortable sensations for a brief period only when you begin to do this.

6 There is nothing to be gained by gritting your teeth determinedly. It is important to explore gently and with a strong sense of kindness. If your attention is pulled away from the body by thoughts about what is arising, simply acknowledge those thoughts and redirect your attention to the body or the breath.

7 You don't need to spend very long doing this practice informally as you go about your day. It can take just a couple of minutes. Try it regularly with other small irritations.

8 When you have some experience and feel comfortable with this practice, experiment with how it feels in more difficult situations, such as not being able to fall asleep. Try to let go of wanting to fix or change your experience, since that is counterproductive. This practice is about learning to accept things as they are—even when we don't like them.

You and Your Phone

The benefits of smartphones are huge—we can stay connected with others regardless of where we are, save time by shopping online, have the latest news at our fingertips—but we can also become enslaved by them. Noticing how you relate to your phone can highlight unhelpful patterns that can impact negatively on your well-being.

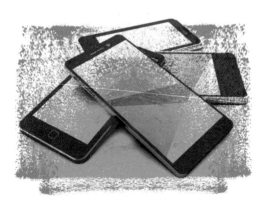

Phone health check

- How often do you check your phone?

- Where are you and what you are doing when you check it?

- What mood are you usually in when you become aware of the impulse (bored, stressed, anxious, calm, happy ...)?

- What you are doing—checking emails (personal or work), social media, shopping, watching videos?

- How long do you usually spend on your phone at any time?

- How do you feel after being on your phone? Does it nourish you or drain your energy?

Remember, you are simply gathering feedback—you would usually do these things unconsciously and so if you can begin to notice the context and the impulse, you can start making more conscious choices. Often it is only minor calibrations that are needed to shift an unhealthy relationship into one that is more balanced.

Technology Detox

The easiest way to tell if your relationship with your phone needs recalibrating is to notice how you feel if you lose it or leave it at home when you go out. If there's a sense of panic or fear of missing out, then things have got a bit out of hand.

Give yourself a break and disconnect from your devices for an hour, half a day, or longer; no emails, no social media, no texting ... How does that prospect feel? The more you resist, the more helpful it will be. Start with shorter periods and choose times when you will benefit from focusing on what you are doing, such as being with friends and family or doing a pleasurable activity.

Technology is there to support us, but it is easy to fall into unhelpful patterns of how we use it. The healthier the relationship you have with your devices, the easier it will be to do this activity. If you find the practice difficult, you probably need to do it!

Social Media: Noticing the Impulse

Notice the impulse to access social media. Explore the moment of impulse without judging. Then, become familiar with the impulse—perhaps noticing what comes before it and whether there are any patterns.

Notice how frequently you access social media. Notice if this varies according to your mood. Simply bring the moment of impulse into awareness.

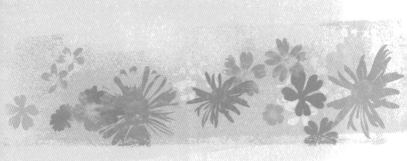

Being With Others

Practice being fully present with others. Avoid checking your phone while in conversation. Notice whenever your mind wanders and bring it back to being here right now. Repeat! What do you notice?

It often happens that when we are with others, we are present in body, but our mind is miles away. Notice what it feels like when you are with someone who is mentally far away. Practice being fully present with family, friends, colleagues, and strangers. Experiment and notice how it affects your relationships.

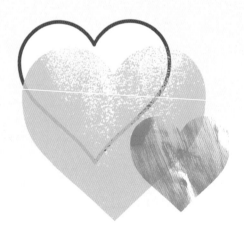

Check it Out

This is a helpful mantra to remind yourself to check in with yourself throughout your day. Just tell yourself to "check it out": where are you, what are you doing, what are you thinking, how are you feeling? Just be present for a moment, and check it out.

Where are you?

What are you doing?

What are you thinking?

How are you feeling?

Paying Attention
to the Body

Most of us spend much of our lives in our heads. We are disconnected from the body and sometimes have an uneasy relationship with it. Perhaps it is aging and letting us down physically, or it doesn't look the way we think it should; maybe it gives us pain or limits what we can do. The practice on the following page gives us an opportunity to become reacquainted with the body.

It is interesting to notice what happens when you turn your attention to the body. What do you discover? We notice physical sensations, and— importantly—how we relate to them. We usually soften around those we like and tense up around those we don't. This tension can create secondary discomfort as well as physiological problems in the longer term.

In this practice, we begin to learn different ways to respond to physical sensations. Practicing being with strong sensations is an important first step in learning to allow and accept our experience of discomfort, rather than trying to get rid of it.

There are certain familiar themes that are key to this practice. Try to keep them in mind before you begin:

Kindness: It is important that there is a strong element of kindness and gentleness in this practice. There is no point in gritting our teeth and determinedly staying with discomfort. That is the opposite of mindfulness. Instead, we are more interested in moving a little closer to areas of discomfort and hovering around them as we explore them, but pulling back to the anchor of the breath as often as we need to.

The wandering mind: You will find that your attention is always being pulled away from the body into thinking, whether it is about the sensations or about other things or other people, in the past or the future. Whenever you become aware of this, simply acknowledge it and bring your attention gently back to the body. We do this over and over again.

The judging mind: We may notice that we start giving ourselves a hard time: "I should be doing this better." "Come on, it's not rocket science—keep focusing!" That is normal. We acknowledge it—judging is here—and then bring our attention back with a huge dollop of kindness.

Being Present

1 This is traditionally a sitting practice, but you could do it lying down. Either way, begin by checking your posture. Bring your attention to the breath. Where do you notice it most strongly? It may be in the belly or the chest, or around the nostrils and upper lip. It doesn't matter where, but just choose and make that the focus of your attention. Stay with the breath for a few minutes, bringing the attention back when it wanders. (For more detailed instructions on how to pay attention to the breath, see page 67.)

2 Expand the attention to include the whole body. Perhaps notice first of all any areas that are in contact with another surface—this may be a chair, bed, textile, skin ... Explore how that feels in terms of texture, temperature, and sensation, noticing differences and similarities. Become aware of how you relate to whatever is arising—is it pleasurable or unpleasant? Perhaps it is neutral. Simply notice how that manifests in the body.

3 Notice if there are any parts of the body that begin calling for attention. Be curious about any sensation that is present and try to discover a bit more about it. Where exactly is it? Is it solid or insubstantial? Is it moving or fixed? What kind of shape does the

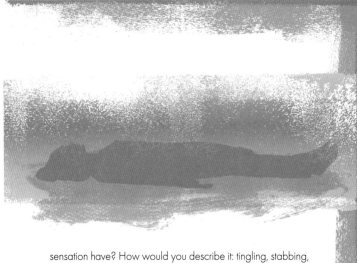

sensation have? How would you describe it: tingling, stabbing, throbbing, needling ...? As long as it feels okay, move your attention in a little closer. We often use the analogy of getting to know someone new, and we want to have a similar attitude of curiosity and interest here, rather than one of analyzing why we might be feeling a particular way.

4 We can also direct the breath, targeting the sensation itself and imagining that we are breathing into and out of that particular area. We are not trying to get rid of the sensation but practicing a different way of being with it—allowing it to be present.

5 If a sensation is particularly strong, it can be helpful to turn the attention to the breath (where you started) and hang out there, occasionally tuning into the physical sensation for a moment or two but returning to the anchor of the breath if necessary. However, taking care of yourself is always the priority, so stop at any time if necessary.

6 We can also move, adjusting our position or "scratching the itch." Ideally, we make a conscious choice to do this and then move with awareness, knowing what we are doing as we are doing it. This is the opposite of the usual automatic scratching or fidgeting that we do unconsciously to get rid of an uncomfortable sensation.

7 Continue for as long as you wish, then narrow your attention to the breath for a moment or two before finishing.

Meditating in this way, whether our focus is the breath, the body, sounds, or something else, shines a light on what goes on in the mind. We notice habitual patterns of thinking and attitudes to ourselves and others. This is all useful feedback. We can start doing something different only once we have become aware of what we might want to change.

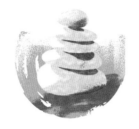

I can make any moment a mindful moment.

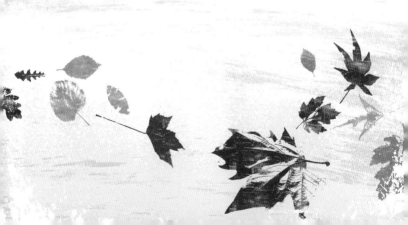

Practicing Quiet

Purposefully making time to be still and calm is wonderfully relaxing. Aim to set aside part of your day, even just five minutes, that is devoted to being quiet—no phonecalls, no radio or TV, no chores. Try to fill silences that do not need filling, and welcome the moments of peace and silence.

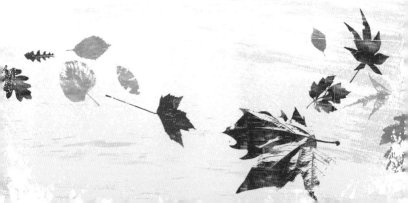

Worrying will never change the outcome. Let it go.

Letting Go of
Negative Thoughts

When things don't go the way we would like them to, it is easy to become trapped in a cycle of negative thinking. This avoidance state of mind is when we don't like the way things are, and we want them to be different. This activates the body's internal stress reaction. Repeated activation doesn't allow time for the stress hormones, such as cortisol, to disperse. Cortisol inhibits new neural branching in the brain and keeps us stuck in negative thinking, and so it goes on.

Our perception of our experience can be positive or negative, and that is something we can influence. We are perpetuating and exacerbating the consequences if we continue to perceive it negatively. We can feed negativity by the words we use to describe something, or by paying it too much attention.

We all fall into unhelpful patterns of thinking from time to time, particularly if we are exhausted. However, the more we practice mindful awareness, the more often we will notice these thoughts as they arise, and it will become possible to see them simply as a transitory mental event rather than a concrete fact:
"Ah, there I go again!"

Letting go of something that we perceive as making us unhappy isn't easy, but it is possible—this is the part of suffering that is optional in the sense that we are feeding it through our thoughts and actions, keeping it "live." Breaking this cycle is one way in which mindfulness has been shown to be particularly helpful.

A New Opportunity

1 Begin by paying attention to the way you describe recent events (either to others or simply in your thoughts). Do you catastrophize or over-generalize, or something else?

2 Once you have noticed the negative thoughts and acknowledged the pattern (without judging it), turn your attention to the body and notice how the thoughts and emotions are manifesting physically. Are you aware of any sensations (perhaps tension or tightening)? Even if you don't notice anything, it is still important to tune in to the body. Name any emotions that you become aware of.

3 If the emotions and/or sensations are particularly strong, you can direct the breath into and out of the area where they are strongest, or simply settle your attention on the breath in the chest (see page 67).

4 You may notice from time to time through the day that your thoughts return to a negative pattern. This is normal, and the instruction remains the same: Notice, acknowledge, and bring your attention to the body and the breath. Repeat over and over!

5 Remind yourself that each day is a new opportunity for things to be different. We can't change the past and we can't predict the future, but we can influence the way we respond to what is arising in the present. We can choose to be with it, even if it feels uncomfortable. We can turn our attention to something more helpful: The breath and/or the body.

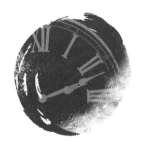

Making time to be
still and calm is
wonderfully relaxing.

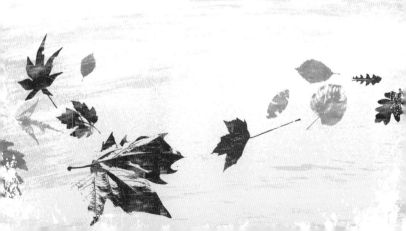

Quick and Easy Aromatherapy

Essential oils have aromatic molecules that pass through the blood–brain barrier. This has a direct effect on the parts of our brain that control our state of anxiety, stress, and sadness. Application of these helpful essential oils to alleviate most negative emotions and moods can be quick and simple. Try the below methods with classic oils, such as peppermint, rosemary, eucalyptus, thyme, bergamot, geranium, and tea tree, to see what works for you.

- **Breathing in relief:** Drop one or two drops of the oil into the palm of your hand and slowly breathe in the scent.

- **Pulse points:** Put two drops onto a cotton ball and gently touch it to your temples and wrists to unwind.

- **Diffuse tension:** Diffusers are popular in homes and offices as they simply emanate serenity. For tranquility when you're on the move, a couple of drops on a scarf around your neck will ease your way.

- **Medicinal mist:** Plug the drain in your shower and turn on the hot water, then add five drops of oil. Let it run for a few minutes, then hop in and breathe in deeply. It is relaxing and invigorating at the same time.

Restorative Incense

Burning incense offers another method of harnessing the power of scent to improve mood and wellbeing. Gentle floral and herbal incenses can aid you in achieving a meditative and contemplative state of mind. Burn any one of them as a stick or cone and you'll hone your "om."

TIP

Incenses such as lavender, sandalwood, jasmine, rose, vanilla, cedar, and lemongrass are wonderful options for encouraging relaxation.

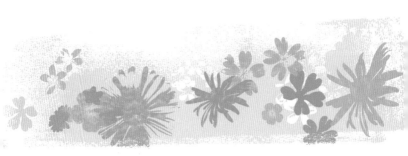

Pause

We often bring our attention to the breath in mindfulness because it is always with us, and directing our attention to the bodily experience of breathing gets us out of our heads and creates some distance from our thoughts. One way to practice mindful breathing is with an ever-so-slight pause between the in-breath and the out-breath, and between the out-breath and the in-breath. Notice the sensations of this liminal moment. Practice attending to the distinct sensations of the in-breath compared to those of the out-breath. Can you experience breathing in and breathing out as two separate events?

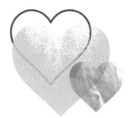

Embrace Today

Today will unfold in its own special way. It's not predetermined, but it's also not fully up to you. Show up with presence, pause before acting, and engage with today the best way you know how.

"To love oneself is the beginning of a lifelong romance."

Oscar Wilde

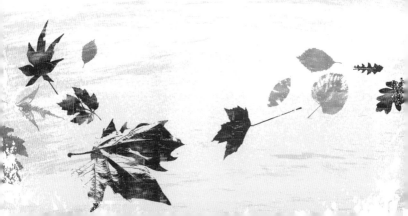

CHAPTER 3

Renew with Time to Thrive

The Benefits of Meditation

The practice of meditation is already well known for helping with a variety of issues we may be familiar with or have experienced ourselves. For example, meditation helps alleviate stress and anxiety, improves communication issues, helps bring greater clarity to our thoughts and actions, strengthens our concentration, increases self-awareness, and helps us to feel more objective about situations that are troubling to us.

The well-being benefits are enough for anyone to think, "I'll give it a go," but what marks this practice out in a world of ever-changing health fads is that meditation quietly works away in the background, ever reliable, and can be picked up with relative ease, without requiring hours of time or even considerable investment.

Meditation doesn't hand you the answers on a plate: rather, it allows you to come up with the answers for yourself. Meditation is like a friend who just sits with you while you come up with your own answers: you inevitably thank your friend for their help when, in fact, you came up with everything on your own. You just needed that space, that inner sanctuary, to discover what you already knew.

Time for You

Taking time out is often at the very bottom of our to-do list; it may not even be a priority at all. It's far easier to relegate our needs to the bottom rung of importance, and yet it is vital that we do pencil in time for our own needs, even if that means taking a few minutes out of our day just to sit and breathe.

Meditation is simply the practice of being in the moment: allowing yourself the time to focus on a singular activity, whether you follow the rhythm and sound of your own breathing, become more aware of your presence and the sensations in your body, or maybe just observe your steps as you take a walk. It is that unique moment in your day when you allow yourself to pause for greater reflection and understanding, which helps calm and declutter the mind. We rarely allow ourselves that time and put enormous pressure on ourselves to be "doing" at every moment, be it working ever-longer hours or making sure we keep up with the current trends and fashions so that the outside is looking perfect, leaving little if not any room for our inner life. You could say that meditation is taking care of the "inner business" of living, helping us maintain a good balance between the inner and outer aspects of our lives.

Count the Ways to Be Kind

We often don't take the time to notice the many ways we can practice self-kindness. Begin to notice what nourishes you—what makes you feel better. Keep adding to the list and begin to intentionally incorporate the suggestions into your everyday life. Pay attention to the simple things that give small pleasures. These are often easier to do than 5-star activities that may take planning and money.

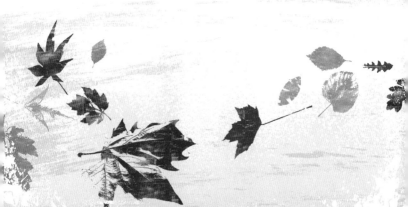

Relax as it is.

Examples of Self-Kindness

- Allow myself to say no

- Slow down

- Acknowledge what I do well

- Have a computer-free day

- Sit in the sun with a book

- Listen to my heart

- Buy some fresh flowers

- Appreciate my achievements

- Encourage myself.

Using Affirmations

When your headspace feels crowded with unnecessary thoughts and your energy is low, taking time to focus on a positive affirmation can help relieve stress, discard unwanted negative energy, and bring focus to the present moment. You can practice this anywhere, at any time.

Affirmation Pick-Me-Up

1 Find a space that is safe and quiet, where you are unlikely to be interrupted or disturbed. Make it as comfortable as possible.

2 Sit down and breathe deeply, inhaling and exhaling through your nose for the count of five. Allow the air to fill your stomach and expand your ribcage and imagine it traveling all the way up to the top of your crown. With each inhale, visualize your breath creating a golden bubble around your body.

3 Repeat the affirmation opposite or adapt it as you wish.

"My intention is to be at peace with myself; eliminate toxic feelings, elements, and energies from my life; unlearn negative and harmful practices and thought patterns; stop checking for people who don't check for me; create space for myself that is nurturing for my personal growth so that I may generate loving energy for myself and for others; nourish my spirit; and balance my energies. I have big dreams and I deserve to live a life I love and let that love radiate, today and every day I grace the Earth with my presence."

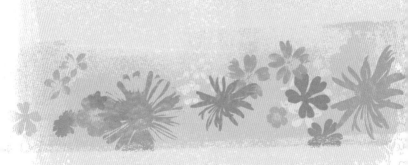

Just Being

Are you someone who is always busy and on the go? How often do you give yourself the gift of time—the time just to pause without any agenda and simply create some space for yourself? Taking a moment and intentionally being still, allowing ourselves to be with whatever is present, is a simple practice we can do at any point, anywhere, for any length of time. How do we do this? The easiest way is to let go of trying to do anything in particular and allow things to be exactly as they are. It's the opposite of "doing," which most of us are experts at!

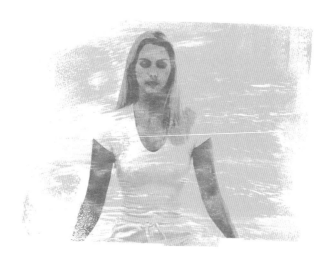

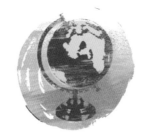

I will focus on
what I can control
and let everything
else go.

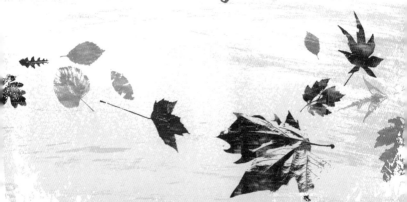

A Loving-kindness
Meditation for You

Take a deep breath and place your hand on your heart. Imagine sending
yourself as much love and acceptance as you can, and silently repeat the
phrases opposite to yourself.

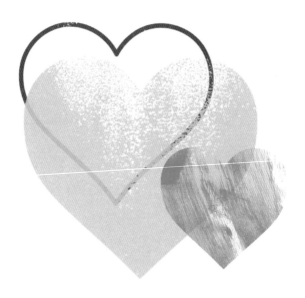

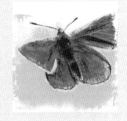

May I be happy.

May I be healthy.

May I be safe.

May I be peaceful.

May I be present.

May I be accepting.

May I be kind to myself.

May I be patient.

May I be curious.

May I be engaged.

May I be hopeful.

May I be loved.

May I be loving.

May I be joyful.

May I be full of life.

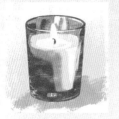

How Do You
Handle Stress?

We all have different ways of managing stress. For the next few days, keep track of the things you do when you get stressed out or overwhelmed—write down the little responses like sighing, or gritting your teeth, as well as the more time-consuming ones, such as reaching for your phone, exercising, napping, or eating junk food. After a few days, consider your list and think about which of your stress responses are working for you, and which ones aren't. Which ones are soothing or energizing, and which ones are agitating or draining? Which ones do you need more of, and which ones do you need less of?

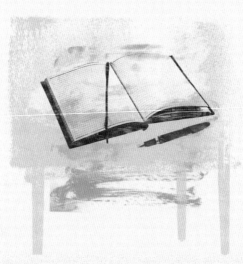

Relax Your Face

Sometimes when we are stressed, it shows up in our bodies without us even realizing it. This simple exercise will help you to become mindful of any tension you hold in your face and help you relax. Take a deep breath and bring your awareness to your face. Unclench your teeth and allow your jaw to relax or even drop open. Soften the muscles around your mouth. Release any holding in your cheeks. Soften your eyes; unfurrow your brow. Feel your breath gently entering your nose, and then gliding over your lips as you exhale. Allow your entire face to be soft and at rest.

TIP

Your eyes take in so much information and stimulation throughout the day—and they need a break. Take a minute to close your eyes and notice what it feels like to give your vision a rest.

Renew with Laughter

Do you remember what it feels like to shake with uncontrollable laughter; to feel consumed by the joy of a single moment, shared with someone you care about or can have fun with? Laughter wipes away tension in a single breath and turns a frowning face into one that is alive and beautiful. It doesn't take much to trigger a giggle: just thinking about something funny that has happened in the past can provoke laughter and increase happiness. Phone a friend, tell a silly joke, or read a favorite cartoon strip; look for the absurd in every situation.

TIP

The media focuses on drama, death, and destruction, but you can make your focus good news only. These events might be small milestones, such as a ripening of a long-awaited homegrown tomato, a dog that was lost now found ... it doesn't matter what, as long as you perceive it as good news! Reflect at the end of the day on what you notice in the head, heart, and body.

Becoming Happy

The good news is that you don't have to be happy to become happy.
The moment you begin to smile, laugh, relax your shoulders, and wipe away
the furrowed brow, two interesting things happen:

• The brain responds by releasing endorphins, which are the attraction
hormones, and oxytocin (the "cuddle" hormone), making you feel instantly
more positive, relaxed, and attractive.

• Those around you will behave more positively.

The result is that the brain learns to become happy, even if you didn't feel that
way to begin with. Practicing this secret of happiness over time will see you
through tougher times and carry others with you.

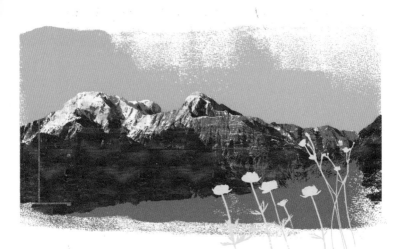

"Keep on knocking,
and the joy that is
inside you will find a
window and look out
to see who is there."

Rumi

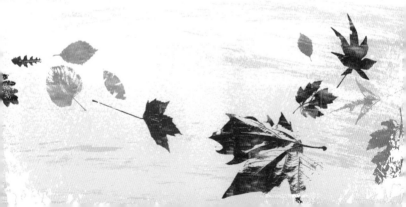

Adjusting Your Posture

When did you last check your posture? Are you often hunched over? Do you slouch when you sit? Get used to checking in regularly with your posture throughout the day. Our external posture often reflects our internal state of mind. Notice the connection between the mind and body. Familiarity with how your posture reflects your state of mind—both positively and negatively— allows you to make adjustments. Consciously sitting tall can help connect you with the strength of your "inner mountain." You can also do this practice while standing and walking. Notice how you hold your head and how this influences your mood. Experiment and see what you discover.

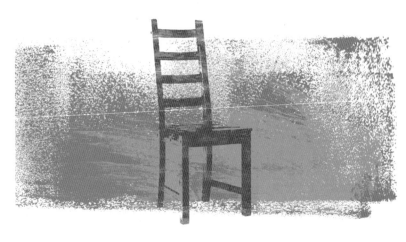

Sitting Tall

1 Sit in a chair with your feet flat on the floor. Imagine a silken thread running all the way up the spine, along the back of the neck, and out through the crown of the head.

2 Give this "thread" a gentle tug so that your spine straightens, the crown of the head lifts toward the ceiling, and your chin becomes slightly tucked in.

3 You are now sitting tall, the lower half of the body grounded and connected to the earth beneath your feet and the torso rising up like a mountain peak.

Daily Stretches

The simple yoga practices on the following pages can be done daily to release stress, improve mobility, promote healthy circulation throughout the body, open up energy in the lower spine, massage internal organs, and aid digestion.

Spinal Flex

This pose is great for anyone who does little to no movement during their day, particularly those who are stuck behind a desk all day or who spend all their time driving. You don't even have to get up! You may do the Spinal Flex as a five-minute break throughout the day.

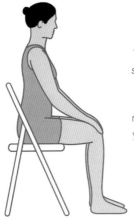

1 Sit in your chair with a straight spine. Place both feet flat on the floor, about hip-width apart. Place your right hand on your right knee and your left hand on your left knee. Your arms should be activated but not stiff.

2 Begin breathing in and out of your nose, filling your belly with each breath and releasing and pushing your navel to your spine. On the inhale, focus on filling your entire diaphragm. On the exhale, try pushing your breath to the back of your throat and down. (The exhale should sound like a hiss). It's okay if you don't get the breath right the first couple of times; with practice, it will come. It is essential to create an internal awareness during yoga, not only to reap the greatest benefits but also to prevent injury to the body.

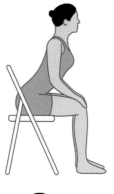

3 With each inhale, arch your spine forward, lifting your heart space upward and pulling your shoulders open and back. Keep your head still and shoulders relaxed.

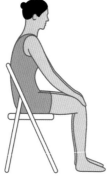

4 With each exhale, focus on pushing the breath out of your body while arching your spine back in the shape of a C. Roll your shoulders forward and tuck your navel toward your spine.

5 Do this five times or as many times as you need to feel relaxed and tension free.

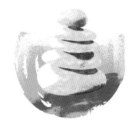

I fully experience
this good feeling.

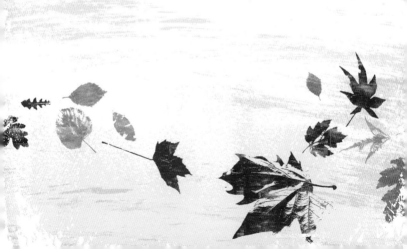

Seated Spinal Twist

Twisting the spine has many benefits. It massages the abdominal muscles and organs, promoting digestion, and keeps the spine healthy. The spine builds up tension between the vertebrae that can cause stagnation and when we twist the spine, we release the hidden tension. This wonderful pose helps move energy downward.

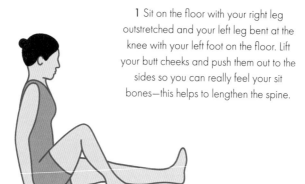

1 Sit on the floor with your right leg outstretched and your left leg bent at the knee with your left foot on the floor. Lift your butt cheeks and push them out to the sides so you can really feel your sit bones—this helps to lengthen the spine.

2 Inhale, raising your arms up to lengthen your spine and twisting to the left toward the bent thigh, compressing your belly against the thigh. Allow your left hand to rest behind you as if it's a support for keeping your spine straight—you don't want to hunch over. Press your right elbow into the left thigh or knee to increase the stretch.

3 If you feel comfortable, turn your neck toward the back of your left shoulder and allow your gaze to follow. Hold for five breaths. Repeat on the other side.

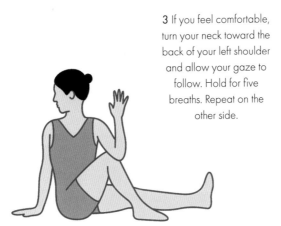

Seated Forward Fold

If you suffer from back pain and intense lower back tightness, one of the easiest methods of relief is a Seated Forward Fold.

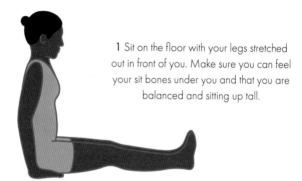

1 Sit on the floor with your legs stretched out in front of you. Make sure you can feel your sit bones under you and that you are balanced and sitting up tall.

2 Inhale, raising your arms up toward the sky and extending them as long as you can.

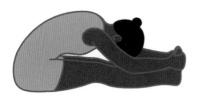

3 On the exhale, lift from your chest and fold forward from your hips toward your toes. Keep your chest lifted to protect your spine; don't collapse.

4 If you can't reach your toes, that's okay, touch wherever you can: ankles, knees, thighs. If this is uncomfortable and your hamstrings are too tight, you can practice this pose using a blanket or yoga block under your tailbone. Hold the pose for five breaths and repeat as needed.

Exploring the Senses

All mindfulness practices are about facilitating that shift from "doing" to "being" mode. A simple way to do this is to use our senses. We can do this practice when we are out and about, at home, or lying in bed.

Sense Awareness

1 Sight: What is in your line of vision right now? Perhaps notice the colors—how light affects a color so that it becomes more than just a hue. Notice how it is made up of multiple tones and even includes different colors. How many different shades of white can you see? How many different colors can you see within white? Name them.

When you are ready, let go of Sight and move your attention to Sound.

2 Sound: Imagine that the body is a radar picking up any sound that comes its way. Each sound is made up of a collection of notes; some make pleasing combinations, but others are more strident and unpleasant. Notice whether there is a physical response to a sound. If you find yourself creating a story about a sound, acknowledge it and let it go. We are simply tuning into the music of the universe right now. When you are ready, let go of Sound and move your attention to Smell.

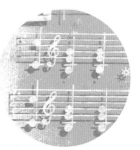

Become aware and be willing to stay with any sense, and see what arises. Sensations may emerge that you miss at first.

3 Smell: Take a deep breath in through the nose. What do you notice? Continue to breathe in and explore scents and smells—liking, not liking, and indifference. When you are ready, let go of Smell and move your attention to Taste.

4 Taste: Become aware of any lingering taste or flavor in the mouth—is there a hint of something? Maybe not. Simply explore, without any expectation of finding anything. When you are ready, let go of Taste and move your attention to Touch.

5 Touch: Become aware of the different textures in contact with your skin. How do they feel? How many can you name? We may experience the touch of objects or clothing, or perhaps the environment—a cold draft against the skin. Become aware of how they may change or of others that come and go ...

6 Finish by taking a moment to become aware of the body as a whole.

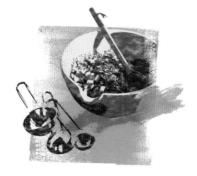

Mindful Eating

How often do you eat while talking to someone, watching television, or checking your cellphone? How does it affect your meal? Do you notice what you are eating—the flavor, texture, smell, and taste? If your attention is distracted, you most likely don't! However, it is very simple to practice something different, and eating mindfully is possible for all of us. It is a straightforward way to move out of "doing" into "being" present in the moment.

The more familiar the "being" mode becomes, the easier it will be to consciously switch between the two modes. Incorporating practices such as this one into your everyday life will make it easier for you to switch consciously at night when you can't sleep, for example.

Many people find that this practice makes their food taste more satisfying and also that they eat less, because they recognize the signs of feeling full sooner than they usually do. However, bear in mind that sometimes what we are eating isn't tasty, and bringing that into awareness won't necessarily be pleasant—and that's okay too!

Enjoy Your Food

1 If you are doing this practice for the first time, you may want to try it when you are on your own. You can do it with a single bite, a snack or meal, or a drink (herbal tea is a particularly good option, because of its strong aroma). You may want to focus simply on the first bite, spoonful, or sip.

2 There is no particular order or steps to follow. We simply pay attention to what we are eating or drinking, engaging the senses—sight, smell, taste, touch, and sound—as we chew, crunch, and swallow. Mindful eating is about savoring your food and drink.

3 There is no need to eat or drink more slowly, but doing so can help to remind us that we are exploring food and drink in a different way from usual. You may notice that a particular smell or flavor brings a memory into sharp focus, which may have positive associations—or not. Simply notice.

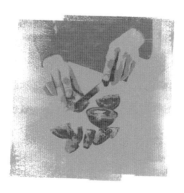

Nourishing Nutrition:
Eat for Energy

To get through a busy day, we all need a brain that is sharp and focused, whether as kids going to school, adults at work, or simply in order to play a fun game of chess with a friend. All day long, the ability to concentrate for a prolonged time can be a challenge, especially as life for many of us is fast-paced and involves ongoing interaction with brain-stimulating technological devices. What we eat and when we eat directly affects how well our brain functions—and that is empowering to know. Our brain needs a steady stream of energy from food for optimal cognition, memory, attention, happy thoughts, and stable mood.

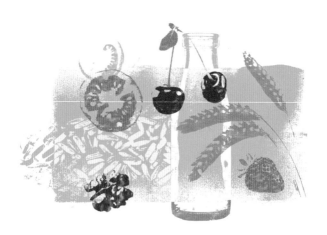

Try to build your diet around foods that provide a large variety of nutrients and brain-supporting fats and oils. Your body needs the best if you are to enjoy a life of vitality, productivity, and joy.

Energy Foods

Top 20 foods for energy, mood, and focus:

- Dark leafy vegetables, such as spinach* and kale
- Purple grapes
- Multicolored berries
- Avocados*
- Coconut oil
- Free-range egg yolks*
- Extra-virgin olive oil
- Wild salmon (smoked, cooked, or canned)*
- Rosemary

- Turmeric
- Gingko tea
- Green tea extract
- Brahmi tea
- Grapeseed oil
- Walnuts*
- Cod-liver oil
- Butter*
- Dark chocolate*
- Navy (haricot) beans
- Pasture-raised meat

Some foods are starred: if you find these foods do not improve your energy, mood, and focus, you may be suffering from a sensitivity to them—consult a health practitioner for advice.

Out of the Ordinary

When we do something that is very closely tied to routine, we are operating on autopilot. When we are on autopilot, it is as if we are sleepwalking. We are unaware of our surroundings, we have no awareness of what we are doing, and we are often wrapped up in our thoughts to the exclusion of all else. However, when we do something out of the ordinary, we wake up, and the body instinctively becomes alert—something new is happening! Our senses become more acute and our experience becomes sharper and more memorable. It's not about making the experience more positive—although often it can feel more enjoyable—but about being willing to step outside of our comfort zone and do something differently.

Memory expert Tony Buzan says that the mind tends to remember things that are different, not things that are the same. So if your routine is unchanged day to day, you will begin to become complacent, because you will no longer notice what you are doing. Making the effort to do things differently occasionally—or swapping responsibilities, or saying thank you with a surprise gesture—will stay in the mind for a long time and have a great impact.

Ways to Change it Up

Use your imagination and come up with something you can do each day that is out of the ordinary. Wake yourself up!

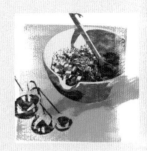

- Take a different route.

- Choose a different seat.

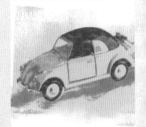

- Cook something different. Eat something different. Drink something different—a different brand, flavor, topping.

- If you usually eat your lunch indoors, try going outside (or vice versa). If you usually read a book or listen to music on your commute, what happens if you simply sit with the experience without any distraction?

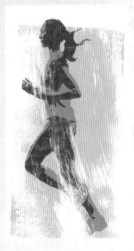

- Make eye contact with people.

- Wear a color or pattern you would normally avoid.

- Shake up your timetable—go to the shops or gym at a different time than usual, or leave the house a few minutes earlier or later.

Just One Thing

Focus on just one thing at a time, giving it your undivided attention. Notice how doing so affects you and also the job at hand. Experiment with different types of tasks, perhaps while you're at work, out shopping, or when you are with other people. What do you notice?

Multitasking is often praised yet it divides attention. This lack of focus is more inefficient because things are missed, and time and energy are lost due to the constant switching back and forth. Continually bringing your attention back to one point helps to develop concentration and focus.

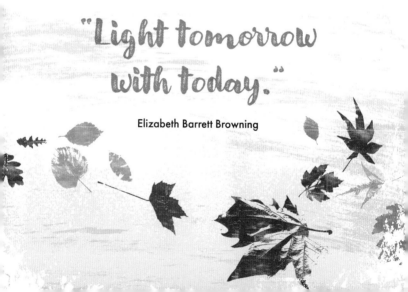

"Light tomorrow with today."

Elizabeth Barrett Browning

Going with the Flow

Mihaly Csikszentmihalyi (pronounced "me-hi cheek-SENT-me-hi-e") has had a huge influence on our understanding of what it means to be happy through his work on a concept he calls "Flow." He is one of the world's leading experts in the field of positive psychology. When we are in flow, we stop feeling conscious of time because we are so absorbed in the task. The results of our work seem to come through us rather than from us. The conditions needed for flow include:

- A sense of being involved in the task.

- A feeling of being outside the bounds of everyday reality.

- A sense of clarity and focus—we know what we are doing and where we are going.

- Taking on tasks that we have the skill level to complete.

- Having the discipline to concentrate on what we are doing.

- A sense of timelessness—of being so involved that we are not aware of time passing.

His work has clarified that for a task to be satisfying, it needs to be challenging, but within the scope of our abilities. If there is too much stress involved, productivity diminishes; if it is too easy, the motivation to do the task drops. Flow is the opposite of apathy—it drives us to act with purpose. When we are in flow, our sense of self is suspended, although completion of the task reaffirms self-value and provides a sense of satisfaction for work well done.

Vanilla Bean Vitality Bath

We often think of bathing as a way of slowing down, but it can also offer a reviving experience, particularly if incorporating appropriate scents. Vanilla is known as an energy enhancer—an excellent combination for feeling more uplifted when you need to.

Whole vanilla bean

1 cup (240g) Epsom salts

4 drops of vanilla extract

MAKES 1 PORTION

Put the vanilla bean into a glass jar with a lid or cork closure. Put the salts into a mixing bowl, add the drops of vanilla extract, and fold in thoroughly with a wooden spoon. Transfer the salt mixture into a jar and let sit overnight while the vanilla bean infuses into the salts.

To use, add the entire contents of the jar as you run a hot bath. Make sure to add the bean pod to the bath, too, for a full dose of high energy.

Tea Leaf Toner Mist

Having this bracingly minty toner on hand will be an enchanting refresher whenever you need it.

2 teaspoons peppermint leaves

2 teaspoons white sage tea

½ cup (120ml) boiled distilled water

3 drops lavender essential oil

4fl oz (110ml) aloe vera gel

MAKES 6FL OZ (170ML)

Place the peppermint and tea leaves into a French press (cafetière) and pour the freshly boiled water over the herbs. Let steep for 10 minutes, then add the lavender essential oil drops. Pour the aloe vera gel into a 6fl oz (170ml) spray bottle, followed by the warm herbal tea, and seal the bottle. Shake well and refrigerate.

Anytime you need to feel restored, spritz the mist on your face, arms, and legs. You will feel refreshed instantly.

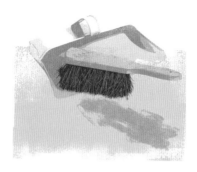

Clearing the Clutter

We need to make space for new things to come into our lives. If it's not lighting you up, start saying no. You don't have to take on projects you hate, deal with people who make you feel bad, or keep doing something just because you're worried that something better won't come along. Start believing in the power of saying no to clear away things that don't feel good to you.

Clearing can mean physically clearing clutter that's dragging you down, or changing the way you approach something—for example, deciding to only check your inbox once a day. It can also bring up bigger things like reassessing your job or relationships and setting up boundaries.

Look at each area of your life and think about what feels good and what feels less than good, and begin making adjustments by saying no or outsourcing what you can. Start small and begin to see the changes that take hold.

Create Some Space

We can fill our days with activities and things to do. When we are busy, we don't have time to pay attention to how we are feeling. If we can consciously create some unscheduled space, we have the opportunity for the unexpected to arise.

Plan to Not Plan

Deliberately create some space in your day for you alone. It may be 5 minutes or 60 minutes. However long it is, leave it unplanned and respond to whatever arises in that period. Notice how it feels before, during, and after. If this feels uncomfortable at first, notice, acknowledge, and stay with it if you can.

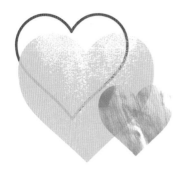

Get Back to Nature

Nature is an instant mood booster. It's revitalizing, and it will help to restore strength and energy levels. Being in a calm and pleasant environment and connecting with the natural world improve levels of serotonin and oxytocin, hormones that make you feel good. When you are feeling low, try taking a mindful stroll through the countryside. Engage your senses as you walk, and take in not only what you can see, but what you hear, smell, feel, and taste. Breathe deeply and let the power of nature infuse you with vitality.

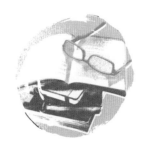

Downtime is your
time. Reconnect
and renew.

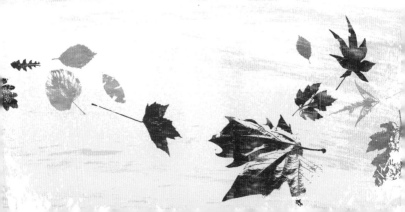

Text credits

© Anna Black: pages 14–15, 17, 18–19, 22–24, 27–43, 61 bottom, 62–63, 67–69, 71, 72, 74–82, 84–88, 90, 92, 102–103, 106, 112 bottom, 116–117, 126–129, 133, 134, 139

© Lois Blyth: pages 61 top, 112 top, 113, 132, 135

© Stephanie Brooks: pages 100–101

© Christine Burke: pages 44–45, 47–49

© Marc J. Gian: page 52

© Cerridwen Greenleaf: pages 50–51, 94–95, 136–137

© Nikki Page: page 70

© Rika K. Keck: pages 130–131

© Noelle Renée Kovary: pages 104–105, 118–125

© Kirsten Riddle: page 140

© Sarah Rudell Beach: pages 16, 54–57, 66, 83, 91, 96, 108–111

© Leah Vanderveldt: pages 10–13, 138

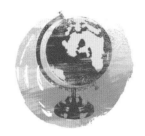

"Take rest: a field
that has rested gives
a bountiful crop."

Ovid

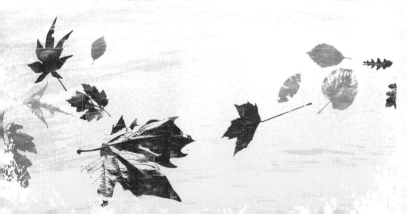